FAMILY EXPLORATION:
PERSONAL VIEWPOINTS FROM MULTIPLE PERSPECTIVES

A Workbook to Accompany
FAMILY THERAPY
An Overview
Eighth Edition

Irene Goldenberg
UCLA

Herbert Goldenberg
California State University, Los Angeles

Arthur Pomponio
National Psychological Association of Psychoanalysis

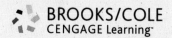

BROOKS/COLE
CENGAGE Learning

Australia • Brazil • Japan • Korea • Mexico • Singapore • Spain • United Kingdom • United States

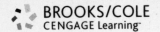

For product information and technology assistance, contact us at **Cengage Learning Customer & Sales Support, 1-800-354-9706**

For permission to use material from this text or product, submit all requests online at **www.cengage.com/permissions** Further permissions questions can be emailed to **permissionrequest@cengage.com**

ISBN-13: 978-1-133-30857-7
ISBN-10: 1-133-30857-0

Brooks/Cole
20 Davis Drive
Belmont, CA 94002-3098
USA

Cengage Learning is a leading provider of customized learning solutions with office locations around the globe, including Singapore, the United Kingdom, Australia, Mexico, Brazil, and Japan. Locate your local office at: **www.cengage.com/global**

Cengage Learning products are represented in Canada by Nelson Education, Ltd.

To learn more about Brooks/Cole, visit **www.cengage.com/brookscole**

Purchase any of our products at your local college store or at our preferred online store **www.cengagebrain.com**

Printed in the United States of America
1 2 3 4 5 6 7 15 14 13 12 11

CONTENTS

NOTE TO INSTRUCTORS

This workbook is designed to help students understand family therapy theory and practice by applying the principles and concepts to their own lives. We hope to stimulate students to think about themselves in the context of the family in which they were raised and to consider how those earlier experiences affect their current relationships. When carried out conscientiously, the exercises in this workbook should prove to be a profoundly moving and fruitful experience for students and instructors alike.

We've compiled over 300 questions, plus some class exercises, divided according to chapter topics in our text (Family Therapy: An Overview, 8th edition) and further divided by topics within each chapter. In our experience, most instructors find it useful to select a specific set of questions, depending on their judgment of relevance to their teaching goals, rather than asking students to answer every question. While we've tried to reduce redundant questions, sometimes answers may be repetitious. Should this be the case, students should be encouraged to pick other questions that avoid redundant responses. In our opinion, students should be allowed to skip questions that, for personal reasons, they wish not to answer.

Since honest responses to the questions can be self-revealing, students should be encouraged to keep the material confidential while they fill out this workbook, treating it as one would a personal journal or diary, and not sharing answers with family members or fellow students as they go through the process. If material arises that proves painful or difficult, and beyond what would be appropriate for instructor-student dialogue, the student should be encouraged to seek professional help, preferably utilizing a family therapy mode, as appropriate.

Irene Goldenberg

Herbert Goldenberg

Arthur Pomponio

PREFACE

This workbook is intended to help teach you about the theories, viewpoints, and perspectives of family therapy by encouraging you to examine your own family experiences. We believe the theoretical material will come alive and the entire learning experience will be enhanced and become more meaningful as you begin to see how these concepts apply to your own family experience. We've provided what we hope are a series of stimulating questions to start you thinking about family life. The more effort you make, the more you will get out of the exercises. Your instructor will likely select those questions she or he deems most important in maximizing your learning experience.

All families tell stories about themselves. We Millers love to argue; we Salingers adore children; we Changs have great memories; we Avilas are mathematically inclined. Typically such stories are passed along over generations and are adopted, often without challenge, by new generations. You undoubtedly have your own set of family stories heard from parents, grandparents, and other relatives.

Sometimes such stories are passed down as problems that require attention. The Peterson men are mean and self-centered. The Washington women always get involved with the wrong men. The Hardys have always been hard drinkers. The Smiths cannot take pain.

We would like you to use this workbook to investigate the stories your family has agreed to tell about itself—especially how these stories affected the adult you became. Through a series of exercises, we hope you will scrutinize the myths and legends, truths and half-truths, realistic self-appraisals and self-deceptions, strengths and resiliency that exist in your own family, all in the service of aiding you in understanding many of the beliefs with which you grew up and which influenced your personal development. Understanding yourself and your own family experience will profoundly help you in your work as a family therapist. Should you require extra space beyond what we have provided in answering a question, simply insert additional sheets to complete your response.

If, as you proceed through these exercises, you find that you require further assistance or clarification, refer to Family Therapy: An Overview, Eighth Edition, by Herbert Goldenberg and Irene Goldenberg (©2013). (The exercises in the workbook are organized according to the chapters in the text.) You can also refer to the original sources, listed in the Reference section of the text, for more detailed reading.

To gain the most from this workbook, you must be honest about yourself and your family. At times some of you may feel the questions are too personal, too exposing, too upsetting; those questions can be skipped. Ideally, however, this will rarely if ever be the case, and the workbook experience will act as a catalyst in your personal growth process. It may also serve as a vehicle for finding your strengths and weaknesses, comfort zones, and blind spots, as a potential family therapist. Don't hesitate to share self-observations and insights, when appropriate, with professors, supervisors, therapists, parents, or significant others. (You also have the option, of course, of keeping the material confidential.) Should you develop "stuck places" or become troubled by patterns you discover about yourself, seek help from someone who thinks in systems terms, understands behavior emerging out of a family context, and who therefore speaks your language.

By learning more about yourself, especially by adopting a family perspective, we believe you can help others, future clients, see themselves within the context of their family lives.

Irene Goldenberg

Herbert Goldenberg

Arthur Pomponio

CHAPTER 1

Adopting a Family Relationship Framework

Family Systems: Fundamental Concepts

1. Entrance into a family occurs by birth, adoption, or through marriage or other committed relationships. Compare the characteristics of family membership (loyalty, support from others, closeness) of two people in your family, each of whom joined the family by different routes. How are they different and how are they alike?

2. All families indoctrinate new members (children, in-laws) into their systems. Sometimes these efforts to forge group cohesion can be felt as pressures against individual wants and needs. Identify three ways your family typically tries to indoctrinate its children into the system (consider your own experience as a child). How have you experienced these influences? Have you ever tried to rebel? How do you join others in trying to similarly influence new members? How do you interact with new members differently?

3. In what type of family structure did you grow up - intact, one led by a single parent, stepfamily? Has divorce of a family member or members played a role in your life? If so, describe the impact of divorce on your experience. How have you been affected by family members whom you think *should* divorce but haven't?

4. What are the expectations you have about the family structure you will be part of in five years? Twenty years? Forty years? Try to frame your answer around a discussion of your attitudes toward marriage, children, divorce, and extended families.

5. Can you think of any special internal stresses that depleted the family's resources as you were growing up? Consider financial downturn, migration, chronic health problems, or the death of a family member. How did the family cope? What community support, if any, was available?

Family Structures, Narratives, Roles, and Patterns

6. Shared family rituals help insure family identity and continuity. List some of the rituals you recall in growing up. Comment on the place and influence of those experiences in your later life.

7. Families typically develop rules that outline and allocate the roles and functions of its members. Those who live together for any length of time develop repeatable, preferred patterns for negotiating and arranging their lives to maximize harmony and predictability. Identify and describe the roles that you played as you grew up. Which stayed the same over time and which have changed?

8. Most families have an outlook that perceives the world in general as a positive and predictable place or as a dangerous and menacing one. This perspective affects all family members. The stories that the family tells about its outlook are part of its narrative. Describe the narrative of your family's worldview. Did it change over time? How were you affected?

9. Draw a picture of your family. Be sure to include all members. When you have finished, note what you see about your view of relationships, alliances, and coalitions in the family.

10. List in order of importance the roles that you currently play (son or daughter, friend, student, lover, neighbor, etc.).

1. _____   4. _____

2. _____   5. _____

3. _____   6. _____

Which of these roles are integral to your sense of self (ones you believe you cannot do without)?

Of all the roles listed above, which one would you insist on holding on to most strongly?

Of all the roles you have listed as currently playing, which would you find it easiest to give up?

Resiliency

11. All families face challenges: an unexpected death, the divorce, job loss, retirement. What resiliency factors were available in a challenging situation in your family? How did the family reorganize itself, solve problems, and cope with threat?

12. Family resiliency can be a function of intact support systems: networks of friends, extended family, religious groups, community resources. Can you identify the support systems that helped your family in a crisis?

13. Identify an experience that severely tested your family's resiliency. Were you able to recover? If so, what resources, from both within and outside the family, were you able to call on to help? If not, what do you think might have helped your family to cope more effectively with the experience?

14. What role did spirituality play in your family life when you were growing up? Did you receive guidance or comfort from a religious community or other groups with strong religious components in their teachings? Comment on their impact on your current views about religion and spirituality.

Gender and Cultural Considerations

15. Family systems are embedded in a community and in society at large. Which of the following social or cultural factors do you believe were especially significant in your family of origin? Choose one or more and elaborate.

Race	Sexual Orientation
Ethnicity	Religious Orientation
Social Class	Immigration Status

16. Cross-cultural and cross-racial adoptions are more common today than in years past. How would these phenomena have been viewed by the members of your family twenty years ago? How are they viewed by them today? Compare past and present views and describe the changes to the family system that might explain any differences.

17. Describe an incident where you or a member of your family became aware of class differences in an exchange with another family. By examining your own reactions to the incident, describe your own views on class differences.

18. What were the messages about work and gender roles you received growing up? Did your mother work outside the home? How were home chores divided? What was your father's role in childcare? If you have siblings of a different gender, were you treated differently because of the different gender status? If so, how?

19. How would you describe your own ethnic background? Describe some influences on your values, attitudes, and present behavior that can be attributed to that background.

20. Provide an explanation of some behavior of yours that has been criticized by a significant family member - first in the language of linear causality and then in that of circular causality.

21. Consider a problem that exists or has existed in your family (say, an adult's drinking problem, or chronic unemployment of a parent, or a child who is a slow learner or one who refuses to go to school.) Describe the problem as it is understood by your family.

Now rethink the problem as a possible product of a flawed relationship between two or three members. Do you play a role in this problem? Describe the various flawed relationships.

The Identified Patient

22. At different stages of a family's life cycle, different members may be labeled the "identified patient" or the symptomatic person. Did this occur in your family? Who was so designated? Did you ever receive that designation? How did it affect your everyday behavior and your picture of yourself? How do you imagine this designation affected a different family member?

23. Is there currently an identified patient in your family, perhaps labeled "sick" or "bad"? Does this person drain off tension for the family, or distract from other underlying problems? If so, identify the underlying problems. How have you reacted?

How did this designation get established? How could it be changed?

What would happen to the interaction of the remaining family members if this person left?

CHAPTER 2

Family Development:
Continuity and Change

Developing a Life-Cycle Perspective

24. Developmental tasks refer to those activities or experiences undertaken by families to overcome conflicts that need to be mastered at various stages in the family life cycle thus enabling the family to move to the next developmental stage. Identify an important family problem. What steps did your family take to overcome it? How did your family change once the problem was overcome?

25. Think back to when you were first married or initially entered into a significant romantic relationship. Did your sense of your independence change? Did your partner's? If so, did these changes cause problems in the relationship? Were you able to overcome the developmental challenges that accompany partnering? If so, how? If not, why not?

26. In a marriage, each spouse usually acquires a set of roles and adheres to a set of rules, often unstated, for marital interaction. In your parents' marriage, do you believe these patterns enabled each individual to maintain a separate sense of self? Elaborate.

27. After successfully weathering an important developmental transition, how did your family reset its priorities? Identify the situation and describe the changed priorities.

28. How flexible would you say your family is in meeting stresses and developmental transitions? Describe the difficulties your family typically experiences in facing transitions. What are its strengths?

29. Both continuity and change characterize the family system as it progresses through time. In some cases the changes are orderly, gradual, and continuous; in others they may be sudden, disruptive, and discontinuous. Describe a long-term change (such as reacting to a child's changing behaviors through her or his adolescence or coping with a chronically ill family member) that took place (or is taking place) in your family. How does your family process long-term transition? Or does it? Does your family seem capable of processing the associated stressful experiences? What problems have emerged when family processing seems to have stalled?

30. What gains and losses occurred for each family member (including yourself) when you first left home?

31. The stress on the family system during a transition may actually give the family an opportunity to break out of its customary coping patterns and develop more productive, growth-enhancing responses to change. Identify a situation in which your family left old coping patterns and developed more growth-enhancing alternatives.

32. Are there any single-parent-led families in your extended family? How did solo parenting come about (divorce, widowhood, abandonment, adoption, etc.)? Are there particularly noticeable characteristics (economic hardship, fatigue, role overload, etc)?

33. What were the critical transition points for your family of origin (e.g., marriage, birth of first child, last child leaves home)? Were there one or more points of particular crisis involving the resolution of any of these tasks?

34. Describe the vertical and horizontal stresses around a crisis time in your family (death, illness, financial setback, moving to a new location).

35. How did the cultural background that each of your parents brought to their marriage blend or conflict with one another? What were the major consequences for the children?

36. In many families, adolescents are the focus of much attention, as if they and not the family system are the basis of family conflict. What was going on with your family members at the time of your adolescence that contributed to family harmony or disharmony?

37. Describe the stage of life your parents were in when you reached adolescence. How did this affect your adolescence?

38. Will you or have you left your family's home to live alone or with others? If so, how did your mother and father react to this stage in family development? Were their responses different from each other? How?

39. At what age do you think it is appropriate to get married? How have your background and family experiences shaped your attitudes toward marriage and its appropriate time in your life?

40. Assuming you are old enough, think back to your late adolescence, emerging adulthood and young adulthood. How would you characterize your developmental changes through these stages? Did your family notice and react to your changes? How?

41. Do you know of a marriage where a new spouse had difficulty gaining entrance into the family circle of their marital partner? What personal and family problems derive from such circumstances?

42. How often should a newlywed couple visit or talk by telephone with their parents? How has your background shaped your thinking?

43. Many traditional-aged students attending sleep-away college today are in continuous contact with their parents by phone, email, text messages, and digital social networks. As a general rule, do you think this much contact between student and home is healthy, unhealthy or is the question of health irrelevant? How might such activity help the student to achieve developmental tasks and how might it hinder those achievements? Use your own situation, if appropriate.

44. Have you personally witnessed the arrival of a child disturb the family equilibrium of a previously well established but childless couple? How? How did they cope with the imbalance? In what ways did husband and wife react differently? Did grandparents reenter the family system?

45. Have you experienced the death of a grandparent? Was it the first death where you were involved? How did the family handle it? What reactions of yours do you recall?

46. Overall, how has your family dealt with life cycle transitions? Did they deal with job changes, children leaving home, marriages, illness or death of family members with the same equanimity? Can you remember a transition that was problematic for the family? Was the family "stuck" for a period of time? How, and how well, did they move beyond the impasse? Are there residual consequences today?

47. Consider the issue of stress in your family. Did the stress first appear in your parents or grandparents? Were family patterns (e.g., drinking), attitudes (all the men in this family are weak) or secrets (grandma and grandpa never actually got married) passed on to you? What has been their influence on your outlook and expectations?

26

48. Consider how you and your family experienced your sexual development through adolescence and into emerging adulthood. Did you feel understood and supported? Describe how you experienced your family during this period of your life.

49. Did you ever live in a single-parent-led family? If so, what were the significant consequences for the family (economic hardship, grief, loss of a support system, etc.)? Were there any family resilient factors that emerged?

50. From your own experiences, or just from speculation, what do you think would be the major family problems in a joint custody arrangement?

51. Have you known anyone raised by a gay or lesbian couple? Can you describe the family relationships during early childhood and during adolescence? Did you observe any special problems in this family structure?

52. Was there someone gay or lesbian in your nuclear or extended family when you were growing up? Was his or her sexual preference out in the open or was it kept secret? How did it affect your family? If you are the gay or lesbian person, how did your family react to your experiences as you grew up?

CHAPTER 3

Gender, Culture, and Ethnicity
Factors in Family Functioning

Gender Issues

53. Which of your parents played a more nurturing role in raising their children? Did this activity have high or low status in the family?

54. You often hear the phrase "It's a guy's thing." Discuss a recent incident you have experienced where gender might have provided an explanation for the behavior.

55. How do you experience women who are assertive and driven and men who are passive and emotionally vulnerable? Take an honest assessment of your views. How might your thoughts and feelings influence your work as a therapist?

56. Did you grow up with same-sex or opposite-sex siblings or both? Where were you in the birth order? How did these experiences affect your attitudes regarding gender issues?

57. How was power distributed in your family? Who was in charge of what? What role did gender play in forming these assignments? What happened within the family if one member tried to step outside of their assigned gender role?

58. Did you experience directly or hear about domestic violence growing up? How did you react? What impact has the experience had on your current primary relationships? Whether from direct experience or from general awareness, does knowing the gender of the perpetrator and victim influence you in terms of your gender views? How? How might your views on gender and violence affect your work with female clients? Male clients?

59. List in two columns the values that had the highest and lowest valences in your family of origin. Include the following (and any others you wish to add) in your list.

Autonomy   Relationships
Nurturance   Dependency
Control   Caretaking
Independence

HIGH VALENCE   LOW VALENCE

_____   _____
_____   _____
_____   _____
_____   _____
_____   _____

60. Did your family approve of your behaviors in terms of gender? How did their approval or disapproval affect you?

33

61. Name and describe some ways in which a gender-based rule or sexist attitude or stereotypic sex role assignment affected the kind of adult you became.

Gender, Work, and Family Life

62. Did your mother work outside the home? How did that affect the distribution of power in the family?

63. Did your father ever lose a job or suffer significant economic loss? If so, how did it affect him? Did it affect the distribution of power in the family? If so, how?

64. What kinds of toys were you given as a child (e.g., dolls, trucks)? Did you play with them under a gender schema of what was considered masculine or feminine? To what extent did such play enhance or inhibit your development from a gender perspective? What kinds of toys will you give your children? Why?

65. What strengths, if any, have you acquired by bypassing traditional gender roles? Any special enjoyments from breaking the rules? Any significant mishaps?

66. To what extent do the following qualities stereotypically attributed to men characterize the men in your family? What were the consequences to your developmental experience?

    (a) an *antifeminine* element, in which young boys learn to avoid in their own behavior anything considered feminine

    (b) a *success* element that values competition and winning

    (c) an *aggressive* element, physically fighting when necessary to defend oneself

    (d) a *sexual* element, the belief that men should be preoccupied with sex

    (e) a *self-reliant* element, calling for men to be independent and self-sufficient and not to seek help from others.

67. Are there specific groups around whom you feel uncomfortable (gays, welfare recipients, transsexuals, child molesters, wife batterers, religious groups)? As best you can, trace the origins of those feelings.

68. Draw a cultural genogram extending over at least three generations, charting your family's social, racial, religious, and migration history.

69. Did you grow up with people culturally and ethnically like yourself? If so, how did that contribute to your stability and sense of belonging? If you grew up in an environment where you felt different, how did that affect your sense of yourself and your acceptance by others?

70. Which social class best describes the one in which you grew up? (Circle one)

Working class   Lower middle class   Middle class
Upper middle class   Upper class

How does this background affect your attitudes regarding class differences? Are there areas in your thinking that might affect your ability to work therapeutically with members of classes different from your own?

71. When and under what circumstances did your family immigrate to this country? How did this event affect your current attitudes regarding immigration of others?

72. Family therapists must try to distinguish between a client family's patterns that are *universal* (common to a wide variety of families), *culture-specific* (common to a group, such as African Americans or Cuban Americans or perhaps lesbian families), or *idiosyncratic* (unique to this particular family) in their assessment of family functioning. Identify patterns in your family that seem universal, culture-specific and idiosyncratic. Identify any conflicts among these patterns and describe how they affected you.

73. Describe how it might feel if you, as a member of the racial or ethnic majority culture in your area, work as a therapist mostly with minority populations. Or, how do you think that you, as a member of a minority working mostly with people from the majority culture, will feel. Identify potential obstacles and opportunities that you imagine will be unique to you.

74. Describe your family's economic status. How has that status affected you view yourself and other people?

CHAPTER 4

Interlocking Systems:
The Individual, the Family, and the Community

Family Systems and Rules

75. Did your family ever move from one community into another with very different social, economic, and cultural characteristic? If so, identify and describe an enduring change in your family experience that resulted from the move.

76. All families have certain unspoken rules, such as: no discussion of sex; deny mother's drinking; never raise your voice; if you can't say anything nice, don't say anything at all. What were some of the rules in your family of origin?

77. What rules did your family of origin have about the position of children both at home and in the community? Did these rules have more to do with custom or tradition or were they based on characteristics of your specific family?

78. Think of an important rule within your family of origin that applied to you (for example, girls are to behave passively) Did this rule and the behaviors associated with it cause you any difficulties as you matured and started to form your own relationships (for example, a girl striving to behave passively frustrates a husband who would appreciate a more assertive woman)? Identify and describe any conflicts and analyze how (or if) you overcame the conflicts.

79. A "marital quid pro quo," in which one partner in a relationship gives something to the other in exchange for something else, is present in all couple relationships. Can you recount some of the marital quid pro quo experiences your parents established? What about the rules in your current relationships?

80. According to Jackson, family members interact in repetitive behavioral sequences (the redundancy principle). Can you describe some significant, recurring patterns in your family of origin? Looking back, can you see how these recurring patterns limited your family in terms of the options it had at its disposal to address issues and problems? Identify and describe a recurring behavioral pattern and the limits it imposed on your family.

81. Scapegoats within a family go under many guises. Do you recognize any of these in your family?

____ idiot   ____ mascot   ____ wise guy
____ fool   ____ clown   ____ saint
____ malingerer   ____ black sheep   ____ villain
____ imposter   ____ sad sack   ____ erratic genius

Describe the behavior of one of the persons so labeled. What were the consequences for that individual later in life?

Maintaining Family Homeostasis

82. Homeostasis refers to the family's self-regulating efforts to maintain stability and resist change. Identify and describe one instance from your family life when a return to stability and resisting change was a benefit and one instance when a successful return to stability maintained or introduced a serious problem.

44

83. Crises occur in all families. Some are resolved relatively quickly, others linger. Describe two such situations in your family - one in which homeostasis was restored quickly, another in which resolution was more difficult.

Feedback, Information and Control

84. How do you signal for attention with someone you care about? Verbally? Nonverbally? Is this tactic different or the same one you used as a child?

85. Recall your adolescence. How did positive and negative feedback experiences throughout your adolescence support or impede or your development?

86. Trace the feedback loops that occurred after a misunderstanding between two members of your family. Was the subsequent exchange of information used to attenuate or escalate the problem?

87. According to the text, family stability is actually rooted in change. Identify and describe a time when your family, called upon to cope with change, found it difficult to do so, creating instability and introducing a new set of problems.

Subsystems, Suprasystems, and Boundaries

88. Identify and describe the important subsystems of your family. Were they organized primarily by generation, gender, alliance against another family member or faction, or by a similar dimension?

89. Identify the different subsystems you belonged to within your family of origin. Describe how your needs, expectations, and behaviors with one subsystem conflicted with those of the other subsystems. How were you affected?

90. How permeable was the parental boundary when you were growing up? What effect did the relative openness or closeness of your family boundaries have on your development?

91. How would you assess the degree of openness of your family or origin? Were the boundaries open to neighbors? Distant relatives? Were your friends welcome or kept at a distance?

92. Sometimes a family will attempt to close a system when they perceive danger in the environment. Under what set of circumstances does your family close its borders? Does stress in the family prompt them to close down or reach out for help?

93. What macrosystems were significant in the life of your family (church, social agencies, health care programs, etc.)? Discuss.

94. Do you recall a time when the school intervened in your family system? Briefly describe the experience and evaluate the effects of the intervention.

95. Depict your family graphically by creating an ecomap. Include the systems with which your family had contact (schools, medical services, churches, community centers, etc.).

CHAPTER 5

Origins and Growth of Family Therapy

Studies of Schizophrenia and the Family

96. Is there someone in your family who has been diagnosed as being schizophrenic or otherwise seriously mentally ill? Describe the reaction to the illness by various family members, and how their reactions affect family functioning.

97. Were any of the following patterns recognizable in your family of origin? Circle one and discuss its consequences for the other family members.

Marital Skew　　　Marital Schism　　　Emotional Divorce

98. The term "emotional divorce," coined by Gregory Bateson, describes the emotional distance or vacillations between overcloseness and overdistance that parents of schizophrenic children often feel as a result of this stressful mental health situation. What examples, if any, are you aware of in your family history?

99. Double-bind messages occur with varying frequencies in everyday life. Can you give an example of such a transaction from home, school, or work where you were double bound? What did you do? What was the accompanying affect? What would have happened had you tried to interrupt the sequence?

100. Analyze some problematic behavior of yours (e.g., nailbiting, smoking, overeating, swearing) from an intrapsychic and then a family relationship perspective. What has changed? Where is the locus of pathology?

101. Describe a family you know, saw on television, or read about in a book in which the members appear loving and understanding, but on closer observation are actually separate, distant, and unconnected. What happens to a child in such a family?

Individual vs. Group Therapy

102. What are your personal attitudes toward group or individual therapy? Which would be better for you? Why?

103. Consider dealing with a problem in your own life from the perspective of psychodrama. Imagine a scenario that reflects your problem. Who would be the "players"? How do you imagine you would feel each time you switched roles and became another character from your problem- scenario?

104. How would you feel about being observed through a one-way mirror as you interact with your family members? Would some members pose or try to be on their best behavior? Would others tend to dominate or control the session? What would your behavior be at first?

Self-Examination

105. If you were a family therapist, which would you be, a conductor or a reactor? Why?

106. How would you feel participating with your family in network therapy in which you would work with friends, neighbors, and employers? How likely is it that you and your family members would agree to this type of family therapy? What might keep you from network therapy? What do you image the benefits might be?

Professionalization, Multiculturalism, and a New Epistemology

107. How comfortable do you imagine you would be working as a medical family therapist having to work with medical personnel in treating families? Can you imagine any difficulties? Identify and describe them. How would it feel to work with patients with serious medical conditions? What support do you imagine you might need to work with these clients?

108. Recount a cherished "truth" about your family that you believed as a child until a family member, friend, teacher, or book author later challenged you to consider whether it was an illusion. What was the impact of the new "truth" on your thoughts, feelings and behaviors?

109. How do you feel about the notion advanced by postmodernists that there is no ultimate truth about anything? How comfortable are you with the constructivist or postmodern idea that every treatment is unique and that no matter what you learn in class, you can not apply learned theories and techniques in the same way from client to client? Identify any negative and positive reactions you have to this view.

110. Has a new person entering your family (a clergyman, a daughter-in-law, a foster child, a visiting relative) helped its members re-evaluate their belief system? If so, how?

111. Reflecting teams sometimes sit in the consultation room while family therapy is taking place, and sometimes observe the therapy behind a one-way mirror. How do you imagine you would feel as the therapist who is being observed by the reflecting team as you work with a family? Knowing yourself, what problems might arise from the knowledge that your work is being examined in this way? Do you feel any benefits? If so, what are they?

112. In your opinion, which is preferable in helping families change: changing their structure or their language and belief system? Defend your position.

113. The Core Competency movement is concerned to help practitioners achieve positive outcomes. How might you reconcile professional expectations for demonstrably positive outcomes with the field's growing interest in postmodern assumptions that there are no ultimate truths? How would you imagine the positive outcomes could fairly be determined and assessed if there are no final truths?

114. Each of us is more than a member of a single group, but rather is influenced by membership in various groups (religious, racial, ethnic, political, gender identification). List, in order of importance, the groups with which you identify yourself.

CHAPTER 6

Professional Issues and Ethical Practices

Licensing Peer Review and Clinical Practice

115. In seeking professional help, what questions would you ask a potential provider regarding his or her training, professional experiences, and licensing?

116. How would you go about selecting a family therapist for yourself and your family? Would you seek out any specific approach to family therapy? If so, which one and why?

117. In working with a family therapist yourself what fee would you expect to pay? Should that fee be more than for an individual session?

118. As a trainee and licensed professional, your work with clients will and should be supervised by qualified professionals. How comfortable do you feel in sharing your work, especially interventions about which you feel ashamed? Will you truly be honest in reporting your work to your supervisors? If not, what about you might get in the way of honest reporting? How might you overcome your personal obstacles to honest reporting?

Managed Care

119. Your family's health insurance is handled through a managed care arrangement. You select a therapist from their provider list, but are told that confidentiality cannot be guaranteed absolutely, since after several sessions the therapist must report details of the treatment to a case manager in order to receive authorization to continue and for you to receive reimbursement. How would you respond? What are your options?

120. As a therapist working with a managed care arrangement, how do you feel about sharing the personal details about your clients with the company's case manager? What will you do if the case manager suggests ways for you to conduct subsequent therapy in order for the company to provide reimbursement? What if you strongly disagree with the case manager's requirement?

121. Is there someone in your family (including you) who would seek psychotherapy if your medical insurance covered the service? What if you need therapy and the insurance does not cover treatment? Discuss.

122. What do you see as the pros and cons of managed care for you and your family? What do you see as the pros and cons of managed care for you as a family therapy provider?

123. If you were seeking family therapy, how important would it be for you to check on whether the therapist's practice was evidence-based? How would you go about finding out? Why is this approach important to you?

Aspects of Professional Practice

124. Your therapist sends you an informed consent agreement prior to starting therapy. Some of the items, such as reporting child or elder abuse, seem unrelated to your problem. How do you proceed in completing the form?

125. Is sexual intercourse between a therapist and client ever justified? Explain your point of view.

126. Safeguarding the personal privacy of the therapist-client relationship has been a cornerstone of individual psychotherapy. Family therapy, in contrast, is sometimes observed or videotaped for later viewing by trainees and supervisors or by professional groups. This brings up the issue of confidentiality. What are your feelings about participating with your family under the conditions of family therapy?

127. How would you feel about sharing your "secrets" with your family members and a therapist? How would you expect your parents to respond to hearing about your secrets?

Maintaining Ethical Standards

128. What are your views regarding therapist record keeping? Would you feel comfortable as a client if the therapist took extensive notes during the session? Brief notes? No notes at all? Explain your answer.

129. Suppose you as a therapist find out from a family that they were seen previously by a therapist who, according to their statements, abandoned them when they could no longer afford treatment. What are your professional responsibilities in this matter? What are your options? How would you proceed?

130. You tell a therapist you are seeing together with your family that you cannot afford his fee. He says not to worry, that he will bill your insurance company as though each member came to see him separately, and the total billing will more than pay for the sessions. Would you agree to this plan? If not, what would you do?

131. What strong religious, political, cultural, or philosophical attitudes or values do you hold that might affect your functioning as a family therapist? Is there any "type" of person you would feel uncomfortable working with? If such a person came to you for treatment, what would you do?

132. A client asks you if what he is about to tell you will be kept in confidence. If not, he adds, he will not divulge the information. Can you guarantee confidentiality? If not, what would you say?

133. How would you, as a family therapist, go about insuring that private information about the family is safely stored in your computer?

134. You receive a call from an adolescent girl in a family you are treating. She asks for a separate individual session this one time. What do you do? Why?

135. A friend of yours, a married woman, thinks she might have contracted AIDS from an extramarital affair, and wants to speak with a therapist but is fearful about the information being exposed. How would you counsel her to proceed? Include a discussion about whether she should use her health insurance policy in this case.

136. A close friend informs you that she had sexual intercourse with her former therapist, and asks you if you think she should tell her current therapist. What do you advise? Why?

137. You and your partner have come for couples therapy. At the end of the first session, the therapist hands you a statement about the duty to warn and about the limits of confidentiality. How would this act affect your decision about continuing therapy?

138. Your therapist tells you he is in his last year of supervision and thus cannot guarantee confidentiality since he must discuss the session with his supervisor. How would you respond? How would your fellow family members react?

139. You must tell a family who has asked that you cannot guarantee confidentiality since you must discuss your cases with your supervisor. The wife reacts negatively and says she will not continue treatment under such circumstances. The husband and two children remain silent. What do you imagine yourself feeling in this scenario? What will you do?

CHAPTER 7

Psychodynamic Models

Freud, Adler, Sullivan

140. In your opinion, should family therapists emphasize the past or present? Explain your position.

141. Psychodynamic models emphasize insight, motivation, unconscious conflict, early infant-caregiver attachments, unconscious intrapsychic object relations and, more recently, actual relationships and their impact on inner experience. How essential do you feel each of these aspects of psychodynamic therapy is to family therapy? Explain your answers.

142. When you hear someone in your family say, "I don't want to hear it" (bad news or something reflecting an interpersonal conflict), they can be said to be using the psychoanalytic defense mechanism of denial. How do you react to someone who not only won't but can not take in difficult of painful information?

143. Most contemporary psychoanalysts no longer maintain the original Freudian view that the therapist and patient are entirely separate individuals with the analyst interpreting the patient's verbal productions from the perspective of such constructs as the Oedipal Complex. For several decades analysts have recognized the importance of the unconscious processes that occur between themselves and their patients that affect the success or derailment of the treatment. What additional responsibilities do you imagine this clinical belief of mutually influencing unconscious dynamics imposes on the analytic/dynamic therapist?

144. How deeply do you think your relationship with your own parents from birth on affected the development of your personality? And how deeply do you think the unconscious aspects of these relationships might affect your work with clients?

The Psychodynamic Outlook

145. Did scapegoating occur to one or more of your family members while you were growing up? What were the consequences of such a role designation? Are there current residuals in that person's relationships to the rest of the family?

146. Do you recognize aspects of either of your parents in your girlfriend/boyfriend, partner or spouse? Why do you imagine you might have been drawn to a person who shares personality characteristics that remind you of your parents?

147. If you presently are in a relationship that has developed problems, would it be better or worse if your spouse or significant other attended the psychodynamically-oriented sessions with you? Explain.

148. How influential have been your parent's conscious fantasies about themselves and their lives been in how you feel towards them? Explain, with examples, as appropriate.

Object Relations

149. Do you know of any special conditions surrounding your birth or early childhood that would have encouraged or discouraged a particularly strong and enduring attachment to your mother? Do you generally feel close, distant, loving, anxious, relatively comfortable, angry, or frightened when you are with your mother? What might the relationship be between how she interacted with you when you were very young and how you experience and understand your personality today?

150. Consider the statement that an individual's capacity to function successfully as a spouse depends largely on that person's childhood relationships with his or her parents. Applied to yourself, what expectations might you have about your own marriage or other long-term relationship?

151. What "introjects" from early childhood are you aware of in yourself today? What impact do such imprints have on your current dealings with adults and children?

152. Does Fairbairn's concept of splitting (the child's internalized image of mother as a good object and as a bad object) shed light on anyone you know who has trouble in forming and sustaining satisfying relationships as an adult?

153. Are you aware of ever having been the target of projective identification (someone close to you projects disowned parts of him- or herself onto you, and then attacked those characteristics)? How did you feel and then respond (or not)?

154. How would you and the members of your family feel about family-of -origin sessions such as those conducted by Framo? What kind of corrective experience might occur?

Self Psychology

155. Describe some early family influences on the growth of your sense of self. Be specific, listing ages and events.

156. Kohut viewed the sense of self as in part emerging from a variety of narcissistic experiences. The well-developed self was mirrored by caregivers in ways that bolstered self-esteem; the less well-developed self might either have been idealized to the point of becoming grandiose or poorly mirrored by caregivers to the point of self-hating, depression, etc. In working with a client, do you think it is your job to mirror your client's self experiences? Why or why not?

Intersubjective Psychoanalysis and Relational Psychoanalysis

157. Do you think the same client could achieve the same outcomes with different therapists? Why or why not?

158. What is empathy? (Hint: It is *not* simly feeling warmly towards someone). How would you as a therapist seek to work empathically with your clients?

159. Do you think that the client could ever deeply, even permanently, affect the therapist? Why or why not?

CHAPTER 8

Transgenerational Models

Family Systems Theory (Bowen)

160. Where do you fit, in relationship to your family, on Bowen's Differentiation of Self scale? Remember that people at the low end are emotionally fused to the family and thus are dominated by the feelings of those around them. At the other extreme of the scale, the high end, people are able to separate thinking from feeling and thus retain autonomy under stress.

Place yourself on the scale below and explain your answer.

1	25	50	75	100
Fusion				Differentiation of Self

161. What scores on Bowen's scale would you assign:

a. your mother?
b. your father?
c. your oldest sibling?
d. your youngest sibling?

Explain your reasons.

162. Would you say that you and your siblings exhibit comparable degrees of individuality? Is one more independent that the other? How does the family as a whole interact with the more independent and more enmeshed member(s)? Explain.

163. How would you rate the degree of anxiety that generally characterizes your family? What happens to the anxiety level in your family when a member seeks to individuate?

164. During one weekly session a husband and wife considering divorce relentlessly express rage towards each other. The therapist invites the couple to bring their sixteen-year-old son to the next session. They therapist asks the young man, "What do you think of your parents getting a divorce?" The boy sadly answers, "Finally, someone has asked me my opinion." The parents realize that they have been so locked in their shared rage that they have neglected their son and not realized the impact of their fighting on him. What is this intervention by the therapist called? How does it work? In the following session, with the young man again present, all three rage at each other with no one hearing what the others are saying. What do you think has happened within the family since last week? Explain.

165. Following the example above (question number 164), the family's college-age daughter comes to the next session. The therapist notices that the siblings seem to want you to tell the parents to get over their problems and to stay together. On hearing this, the parents suddenly join together and attack the children by angrily saying to the therapist: "Whether we stay together or not can't be decided by the children, right?" What has happened to the family system with the addition of the daughter? Has anxiety been moderated by the presence of a new person? Explain the new development.

166. Bowenians contend that any of three possible symptomatic behavior patterns may appear as a result of intense fusion between the parents: physical or emotional dysfunction in a spouse; chronic, unresolved marital conflict; psychological impairment in a child. Did any of these patterns occur in your family? Describe the circumstances.

167. Bowen believed that parents functioning at a low level of differentiation may transmit their immaturity to their most vulnerable, fusion-prone child. Did this or a similar family projection process occur in your family? Which child was most susceptible to such fusion? Explain.

168. Emotional cutoff in a family occurs when one member distances himself or herself from the others in order to break emotional ties. Distancing may take the form of a geographic move, unwillingness to attend family get-togethers, stopping talking to one or more relatives, etc. Has any of this occurred in your family? How did the emotional cutoff affect the problem?

169. Bowen worked with the family in creating a family history (genogram) while Whitaker invited grandparents to join parents and children in a family session. Which would work better for your family? Why?

89

170. Make a genogram of your family, covering at least three generations. What have you learned about relationships within your family from the genogram?

171. Identify as best you can any unresolved attachment issues with respect to your family. If you are aware of any, do you see how they might affect the way you interact with your choice of boyfriend, girlfriend, spouse or partner? Describe and explain.

172. What is your sibling position in your family of origin? How does it match the sibling position of a significant person in your life (spouse, roommate, lover)? How do your corresponding positions growing up affect your current relationship?

91

173. Bowen advocated keeping down the emotional intensity in his work with families, so that the members might more easily think through what was causing their difficulties. Is there a member of your family who plays a similar role? Describe.

Contextual Therapy (Borszormenyi-Nagy)

174. What resources can you find from the past history of your family that sustain or enrich your life today?

175. In your family ledger, what are some of the "unpaid debts" or restitutions that need to be made? If mother worked to put father through school, has she been repaid? Was there an imbalance in childcare responsibilities? Was that debt erased? If not, what are the residuals?

176. Family legacies dictate debts and entitlements. What legacies did you inherit? Were you expected to be an athlete, a musician, a scholar, a failure, beautiful, etc.? How have you carried those legacies into your current relationships?

177. To function effectively, family members must be held accountable for their dealings with one another. How does your family balance entitlement and indebtedness?

178. Has there been a death in your family where you believe grief was never sufficiently expressed? How did that affect family functioning?

CHAPTER 9

Experiential Models

The Symbolic-Experiential View (Whitaker)

179. You and your family show up for family therapy. At first, you all find the therapist to be funny and engaging. In time, though, he starts to introduce his own fantasies and unconscious processes during the session. Once, he even falls asleep. How would you and your family respond to such an approach?

180. Have you ever experienced a time in your life when "acting crazy" was a liberating experience? Describe.

181. Which one of the following two approaches would your family of origin have felt best met its needs: a therapist who believed in dealing primarily with feelings or one who emphasized rational analysis?

182. As a follow up to the question above, would you now pick a therapist consistent with your family of origin patterns or one contrary to them? Explain your answer.

183. How would you feel about having your grandparents (separately or together) in a family therapy session with you and your parents? What special problems would arise? What special advantages might there be?

184. Imagine a situation in which your therapist expresses her or his genuine annoyance with you? How do you imagine you would feel? Could you imagine any benefits to you from this authentic exchange?

185. Whitaker took the position that each person in therapy is, to some degree, a patient and therapist to one another. Discuss your reaction to this statement.

186. How comfortable would you be as a therapist disclosing personal aspects of yourself (your fantasies, impulses, images, or metaphors from your own life) to your clients?

187. Whitaker had a number of "rules" for "staying alive" as a human being and as a therapist, as described in the text. One was to "enjoy your mate more than your kids, and be childish with your mate." Was that rule true of your parents? How true the rule for you if you have a spouse and children? Describe. Why do you think Whitaker believed this rule would help you to "stay alive?"

188. The use of co-therapy as an effective therapeutic technique has been debated. List some pros and cons and state your position. How do you imagine you would feel working with a co-therapist?

189. Read the following dialogue involving a wife, husband, and their therapist. The wife has admitted that she feels despair over the way her husband pushes her around.

Wife: So last night, I made dinner for Bruce (her husband), and after it was all done, he said he wasn't in the mood for the fish I prepared and said he wanted to go out instead.

Husband: I don't see what the big deal was? I didn't feel like fish.

Therapist: What happened?

Wife: It broke my heart to throw out all that good food, but Bruce just wouldn't eat it. We went out.

Therapist. How else did you feel?

Wife: Well, I was ok once we got to the restaurant.

Husband: You wouldn't have known that to look at you. You didn't say a word.

Therapist: I can't stand this! It feels like your husband walks all over you and you are the welcome mat who lets him. I want to punch him out.

Husband: Hey, buddy, watch what you're saying?

Therapist: Why should I? How can it hurt for you to know what your wife feels when you assert yourself so aggressively without concern for her feelings? I'll care about your feelings when you start to care about hers. Do you think you can do that? Can you start to appreciate how it feels to be pushed around?

Can you imagine this sort of interaction ever being appropriate? Following Kempler's Gestalt approach, what would the goal be for this sort of intervention? And again following Kempler, what would you say if you sensed the wife becoming very hurt or frightened or the husband's anger escalating in a dangerous way?

190. Learning to communicate "I" messages is a basis exercise for Gestalt family therapy. For example, instead of an accusatory "You never pay attention to me!" an "I" message might be "I'm feeling ignored by you and it's upsetting me." Talk to a significant person in your life expressing "I" messages only, and note how the transaction between you changes.

The Human Validation Viewpoint (Satir)

191. Satir stressed the mind-body relationship in her growth-enhancing, health-promoting therapeutic interventions. Discuss your own experiences with such body language connections (a pain in the neck, a stiff upper lip, etc.).

192. Satir classified family communication patterns in the following way:

Placater   Super-reasonable   Congruent   Blamer   Irrelevant

Describe a member of your family of origin or your current family using one of these categories, paying particular attention to that person's characteristic way of interacting.

193. Satir contended that the way the family communicates reflects the feelings of self-worth of its members. Dysfunctional communication (indirect, unclear, incomplete, unclarified, inaccurate, distorted, inappropriate) characterizes a dysfunctional family system. Describe your family's communication style and assess the sense of self-worth you believe each member feels and of the family as a whole.

194. Satir contrasted two worldviews with respect to family life: the "Threat and Reward" model and the "Seed" model. Review these concepts in the textbook. Which would you say characterizes the way your family members relate to each other? Provide and analyze an example from actual experience that reflects this worldview.

CLASS EXERCISE

Form a group of four persons in your classroom. Each should choose a new first name, then decide on a last name and assume a family role. Stay with your same sex role, but do not necessarily stay in your real life family (a son can be a father, etc.) Your communication should be as follows:

Pick a communication style and maintain it.

- If you are a blamer, begin each sentence with statements such as "You are never" or "You are always." Find fault.
- If you are a placater, take the blame for everything that goes wrong. Make sure no one gets hurt. Never say what you want.
- The irrelevant one must not communicate in words properly. Be distracting.
- The super-reasonable one must be stiff and proper. Stick to the facts, ignore feelings, or greet them with statistics.

Have a five minute discussion in front of the class. Stop. Relax. Report any messages you might be receiving from your body. What has happened in your new family? How did it make you feel? Share your impressions with one another and with the class.

195. Can you identify any efforts in your family to block emotional engagement (distracting, making jokes, leaving the room, etc.)? What was the result on family communication?

196. What repetitive, negative interactive patterns restrict optimal functioning in your family?

CHAPTER 10

The Structural Model

Structural Family Theory

197. Structuralists contend that a change in the family organization must occur before a symptom in a family member can be relieved. Has such a situation occurred in your family? Who manifested what symptom and what family restructuring helped alleviate the problem?

198. Each family system is made up of a number of interdependent subsystems. Were the key sub-groupings in your family according to age, sex, outlook, or common interest? Explain.

199. Describe the tasks that your family assigned to each of the independent subsystems. How well or poorly do these assignments work in your family? Explain.

200. Minuchin believed that families go through their life cycles seeking to maintain a delicate balance between stability and change. How open to change is your family? Identify the benefits and liabilities that characterize the way your family remains stable or makes change.

201. Are there any conflicts between subsystems in your family that are particularly damaging or destructive to overall family functioning (e.g., older people dismiss what younger people have to say; females believe men are insensitive)? Identity and explain the conflict.

202. Under stress, does your family become more enmeshed or more disengaged? Describe and explain the behavioral consequences for each member of your family and for the family as a whole.

203. Structuralists contend that all well-functioning families should be organized in a hierarchical manner, with the parents exercising more power than the children, the older children given more responsibilities than their younger siblings. How was you're your family of origin organized? What were the consequences of the power arrangements when you were growing up?

204. Some feminists take exception to Minuchin's insistence that a well-functioning family requires hierarchies, arguing that this view runs the risk of maintaining sexual stereotypes. How was your family organized? Was there a rigid or flexible organization? Did it promote sexual stereotyping? What were the consequences of any sexual stereotyping?

205. Do you consider the boundaries in your family of origin to have been clearly defined, rigid and inflexible, or diffuse? What were the consequences on family transaction patterns as a result of such boundaries?

206. The sibling subsystem offers the first experience of being part of a peer group and learning to support, cooperate, and protect (along with compete, fight with, and negotiate differences). How well or poorly did you and your siblings help each other to develop skills in interacting with later peers? If you are an only child, how do you imagine the absence of siblings affected your ability to successfully interact with peers?

207. Structuralists use family mapping to depict a family's structure at a cross-section of time. Using Minuchin's symbols described in the text, draw a map of your family at a particular critical time in its existence, paying special attention to the clarity of boundaries, to coalitions, and to ways of dealing with conflict.

208. Structuralist therapists offer the family leadership, direction, and encouragement to examine and discard rigid structures that are no longer functional and to make adaptive changes in structure as family circumstances and family developmental stages change. Identify a rigid aspect of your family functioning. Knowing your family as you do, explain how that rigidity contributes to family dysfunction. Articulate goals for change. Imagine on behalf of your family what a more functional structure would look like, and indicate the kind of encouragement you feel your family would likely respond to in trying to make positive change.

209. Reframing the meaning of certain behavior can provide a fresh perspective and make that behavior more understandable and acceptable. Reframe the following:

a. Mother pokes into my private matters too much.

b. Father frightens the family when he drinks too much.

c. Sister is selfish and only thinks of herself.

d. Brother gets away with murder because he's the youngest child.

210. How does the reframing in the previous question change your feelings about the troublesome behavior?

211. Structuralist therapists often induce a crisis by introducing anxiety into the family system. They actively encourage family members to interact with each other, often through enactments. The therapist seeks to maintain a therapeutic experience of intense affect and pressure. How compatible are these structuralist goals and interventions with your personality? Explain.

CHAPTER 11

Strategic Models

The Communications Outlook

212. Describe the sorts of relationship definitions (symmetrical or complementary) you tend to get involved in with two of the following groups:

a. your male friends

b. your female friends

c. your parents

d. younger people

e. older people

213. Communication occurs between people at multiple levels. Think of an instance from your own recent interactions with someone close to you that demonstrates how words, body language, tone of voice, posture, or intensity seemed to transmit different meanings Analyze this interaction to see if you can clarify the range of meanings that you were receiving from this person.

214. You have an argument with a friend. Discuss how each of you is likely to punctuate the communication sequence.

215. You are treating a husband and a wife. The husband says that he always pays attention to what his wife tells him about her feelings but feels that she doesn't respect his. She cuts him off and claims that she most certainly listens to what he says and that he should appreciate how attentive she really is. Identify the report and command communications in this scenario.

The Interactional Viewpoint

216. Describe a double-bind situation in which you have been caught. Remember that you must have a close relationship with the person, must respond, and be receiving conflicting messages at two different levels. What did you do?

217. Describe an unsolved problem in your family. What makes the behavior persist?

218. When a therapist tells a client "Don't be in such a hurry to get over your anxiety" what technique is being employed? What is the goal of this technique?

219. A therapist tells a raging couple "Well at least the two of you continue to talk." What technique is the therapist using? To what end?

Brief Family Therapy

220. At what point in your life could you and your family have benefited from brief (up to ten sessions) crisis intervention? (For example, you might consider divorce, death, drugs, alcohol abuse, school separation, or an auto accident as possible crisis times.) Describe the situation and explain why you believe such intervention might have been helpful.

221. A friend has a problem stopping smoking. How would you "prescribe the symptom"? What consequences would you anticipate?

222. Which would feel more comfortable to you as a family therapist: defining the family's problem before the session starts, or getting your cues from their unfolding discussion? Why?

223. You are working with a family that has been struggling to accept that their son is gay. Each week someone in the family discusses how something unkind or dismissive has been said about the son. When you point this out, the mother often says, "We'll have to try harder." How would you, as an MRI therapist respond to the mother? Why?

The Strategic Viewpoint

224. Haley believes that symptoms are indirect strategies for controlling a relationship while at the same time denying that one is voluntarily doing so (e.g., mother becomes ill and can't be left alone when her adolescent daughter wants to go out for the evening). Can you cite an example from your own experiences? As a therapist what intervention might you make to address this symptom/strategy?

225. According to strategists, implicit in every relationship is a struggle for power. What power struggles are you currently experiencing with members of your family?

226. Suppose a friend of yours drank too much and came to you for help in changing this behavior. Can you think of a therapeutic double-bind, a symptom prescription, or a paradoxical intervention to aid in reducing or eliminating the symptom?

227. Describe a current important relationship that you are in, and consider whether a third person is also somehow involved. How does this third person affect the quality or condition of the dyadic relationship? What would happen if the influence of the third person were to become less important or to disappear all together?

228. How would your family respond to a series of directives from a therapist? Would it be easier if he or she were an authoritative expert or a collaborative coach?

229. As a strategic therapist, think of a paradoxical intervention to help a couple resolve issues over jealousy? What impact would you expect the paradoxical intervention to have?

The Milan Systemic Model

230. You finally persuade your family to come for family therapy, hoping the therapist will expose the family "games", which only you seem to acknowledge. Instead, she offers positive feedback on behavior patterns you believe are destructive, and she warns the family about premature change. How would you react?

231. Write a "paradoxical letter" to a member of your family who has refused to join the others in attending family therapy sessions.

232. What were the rituals surrounding the evening meal in your home when you were young? Did you eat together regularly? What topic could be discussed? What topics were off limits and avoided? Did people sit in special places on a regular basis? Who was served first?

233. What circular questioning might be thought-provoking for your family (e.g., "Who first noticed that?" or "Who enjoys fighting the most?")? Write an imaginary script including each of your family members that shows who would say what in response. What is something new that have you learned about your family from writing this script?

234. Choose one of Tomm's reflexive questions to address your family. How do you imagine they would respond?

CHAPTER 12

Behavioral and Cognitive-Behavioral Models

The Cognitive Viewpoint

235. Select a family problem you have discussed earlier in this journal and restate it in cognitive-behavioral terms.

236. Cognitive psychologists pay special attention to how individuals organize, store, and process information. Consider a problem you may have had for a long time, and describe it at these three levels: automatic thoughts, underlying assumptions, and schemas or basic core beliefs.

237. Dysfunctional behavior is said by Ellis to be a result of our flawed or illogical interpretation of the behavior of others. Use the concept of cognitive restructuring to deal with a problem you are currently having with someone. Create a new self-statement.

238. Is there a "negative schema" acquired in your childhood that has been reactivated recently? Describe.

239. Cognitive-behaviorists stress the importance of self-regulation and self-direction in altering behavior. What would be the pros and cons of this approach for you and your family?

240. Describe an incident where you heard one side of a story, then were startled later by hearing the other side. How did you resolve the disparity?

241. Think of a time when you had a long conversation with someone about something important (or, if you keep a journal, look up an entry in which you write about something important). See if you can identify an example of each of the following cognitive distortions. Write down the example, and then consider how you might think differently about what you've written.

a. arbitrary inferences

b. overgeneralizations

c. dichotomous thinking

d. biased explanations

242. Try to shape someone's behavior by giving that person positive reinforcement (a smile, a kiss, a gift, attention) whenever desired behavior occurs, while ignoring undesired behavior. Continue to do so for seven days. Describe your results and draw conclusions.

243. Behaviorists sometimes use the phrase "quid pro quo" (something for something) to describe how couples in successful marriages work out suitable arrangements for exchanging pleasures. Take a look at your parents (or an uncle and aunt), identify an example of a quid pro quo between them and describe the range and frequency of reciprocal positive reinforcements they exchange.

244. Create a "caring days" list with a significant other in your life, of kind actions and words you would like to receive from one another. Be specific in your requests, and ask the other person to be the same. Exchange the lists. After one week, note any changes in the relationship.

245. Were there any surprises in the "caring days" requests you received in the preceding exercise? How did such unexpected requests alter your perception of the relationship and/or change your subsequent behavior?

246. Where did your parents' marriage fall in relation to Gottman's couple schema: volatile, validating, conflict-avoiding? How well did the marriage work? Look at your own relationships. Where do you think you fall in relation to this schema?

247. According to Gottman's findings, and contrary to popular opinion, it is not the exchange of anger that predicts divorce, but rather four forms of negativity: *criticism* (attacking a partner's character), *defensiveness* (denying responsibility for certain behavior), *contempt* (insulting, abusive attitudes toward a partner), and *stonewalling* (a withdrawal and unwillingness to listen to one's partner). Using either your own intimate relationship or that of someone else you know well (parents, grandparents, uncles and aunts, best friend and her or his spouse), identify which form of negativity characterizes each partner. Were the partners able to overcome their characteristic negativity? If so, how?

248. Would a contingency contract have been helpful in resolving any conflicts you may have had with your parents when you were an early adolescent? Describe the problem briefly and set up a contract.

249. Did your parents use informal methods of reinforcing desired behavior (e.g., promising a bicycle if your grades improved significantly)? How well did such methods work? Did they create any problems? Imagine how this approach might help you as a therapist working with clients? Indicate any limitations you can anticipate.

250. Functional family therapists regard an individual's behavior as always serving the function of creating specific outcomes in that person's interpersonal relationships. Observe a friend or family member over several days, noting behavior patterns (without regard to whether you consider them desirable or undesirable), then speculate on the function of the behavior.

BEHAVIOR	FUNCTION
_____	_____
_____	_____
_____	_____
_____	_____
_____	_____

251. Repeat the exercise shown above with your own behavior with respect to your relationships. Speculate on the function of your own behaviors.

BEHAVIOR	FUNCTION
_____	_____
_____	_____
_____	_____
_____	_____

252. Consider a seemingly dysfunctional pattern between two members of your family, but one that nevertheless has persisted. What interpersonal payoffs might exist for the participants that help perpetuate the pattern?

Conjoint Sex Therapy

253. What was the dominant sexual theme transmitted to you by your parents (e.g., sex is a natural and enjoyable part of life; sex is to be endured; sex is not to be discussed)? What has been its impact on your current attitudes toward sex? What attitudes do you expect to transmit to your children?

254. Under what circumstances would you go to a counselor for sex therapy? Would you be expecting psychological or medical interventions?

255. Some sex therapists see couples separately at first, while others start with conjoint sessions. Which process do you think would work out best for you? Explain.

CHAPTER 13

Social Construction Models:
I. Solution-Focused and Collaborative Therapy

Social Constructions

256. How would your mother describe you to a friend in your absence? Would your father agree? If not, how would he describe you? Would a friend concur? What would your friend say instead? How would you describe yourself? What do the different descriptions tell you about how meaning in general and our knowledge of ourselves in particular are created?

257. Postmodernists consider constructions regarding reality to be based on language and communication. Has anyone in your family identified himself or herself, or been identified, as an alcoholic? How did that self-imposed label structure how others viewed and reacted to that person's problematic behavior?

258. Social constructionists and other postmodernists believe that language and culture, which are continually changing, inform how we understand anything, and that there is no final authority on any subject that determines a final meaning about anything. How comfortable are you with this relativist idea in your personal life? If you believe in God as a final authority can you accept postmodernism?

Now consider your comfort level as a therapist with the postmodern position that all meaning is constructed. Do you accept that you and your work with your client create the meaning relevant to treatment instead of meaning coming from diagnostic manuals, information acquired in educational and clinical institutions, and manuals issued by insurance companies? How comfortable are you knowing that you can't learn final truths about yourself as a therapist or about your clients? Will your view affect your work with clients? How?

259. Do you believe in a person being "normal?" Why or why not? If you believe that people can be normal, on what authority do you make this claim? If you don't believe that people can be normal, how would you judge when your clients are "better?"

260. Watch a TV sitcom and choose a character that is at an impasse in solving a particular problem. As a therapist, what might you suggest to help that person become "unstuck"? Does he or she seem to possess the knowledge or resources to get "unstuck"?

261. Different opening remarks by a therapist are likely to set the stage differently and thus elicit different responses from a family. How would your family respond to each of the following?

a. I am concerned to know about your problems. Tell me what problems brought you to see me today.

b. How can we work together to help change your situation?

262. What do you consider to be the advantages and disadvantages of having a five or ten session limit to family sessions?

263. In your family, who would be the visitors, complainants, or customers for therapy? Explain.

264. Can you identify a time when someone helped you re-story your life so that you saw the same events in a new and more positive light? What were the consequences? Did you feel empowered? Did any change feel permanent?

265. Consider someone in your life who always talks "problem talk." How could you help that person engage in "solution-talk"? Give an example and indicate anticipated effects of the change.

266. Answer this version of the "miracle question" for yourself:

Suppose that one night there is a miracle and while you were asleep the problem that you have been worrying about is solved. How would you know? What would be different? What would you notice the next morning that would tell you a miracle had occurred? What would your best friend notice?

267. Emphasizing hope, encouragement, client strengths, and possibilities, solution-oriented therapists believe they empower clients to improve their lives, and in the process help create self-fulfilling prophesies of success. How would a solution-oriented therapist help a family with a severely depressed member who seems unable to feel any hope at all? What do you imagine you will feel if you detect no change within the anticipated five to ten session brief therapy schedule? What might you do?

268. Lynn Hoffman says that "problems are stories that people have agreed to tell about themselves." Write up one of your current problem areas from this perspective.

Now write an alternate story to the above. What has changed?

269. Rate a specific family problem on a ten point scale, with 1 representing the least troublesome and 10 the most. Next, without revealing your rating, ask a family member to rate the severity of the same problem. Compare your scores and discuss the differences in viewpoint your scores reveal.

CLASS EXERCISE

Have a small group of students discuss a problem while the rest of the class, acting as a reflecting team, observes them. Then have the small group watch as the class discusses reactions to what they observed. Reverse the process once again. What did you learn?

CHAPTER 14

Social Construction Models:
II. Narrative Therapy

270. Consider one of the "stories" told and retold in your family. How did its content shape your life?

271. How did the above story become established for you as the "truth?" Do you personally feel it to be the truth?

272. Was there a negative, self-defeating story told in your family as you were growing up? Describe.

273. Assume you are a therapist working from the perspective of narrative therapy. Your client strikes you as a difficult and unpleasant person. You know he has no friends and his family has rejected him. He tells you that he believes that he was born into a cruel world and he is just the product of it. Would you seek to replace this "truth" with a more benign story, such as "it's not your fault," or "the world is neither cruel nor nurturing; it just is"? What might be a more useful and honest way to employ narrative therapy? What narrative might you consider developing instead that somehow still accounts for this man's experience?

274. What has been the "dominant story" in your life?

275. Was a "thin" description of you ever imposed by others (parents, clergy, teachers) in your life when you were young? Were you labeled as bad, lazy, greedy, selfish, rebellious, or something similar? Write an alternative "thick" description of your behavior.

276. Have you kept a letter, a newspaper clipping, a fortune cookie prediction, or e-mail in your wallet? How does such an act relate to your personal story?

277. Describe a primary self-narrative in your life (e.g., "my illness as a child made me introspective", "my grandmother's business success inspired me", "my mother's craziness made me wary of close relationships").

278. Discuss a dominant narrative of your culture (e.g., "a woman can't be too rich or too thin," "men wear the pants in the family," "such and such a group is inferior to us"). How has it affected you?

279. How has society controlled you with its definition of what it means to be a "real man" or "real woman?"

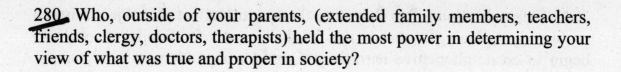

280. Who, outside of your parents, (extended family members, teachers, friends, clergy, doctors, therapists) held the most power in determining your view of what was true and proper in society?

281. Which one of the following political forces has most affected your life: racism, sexism, class bias, or homophobia? Discuss.

282. Externalization often has the therapeutic effect of objectifying a problem and placing it outside the family in order for family members to begin to create alternative narratives. Consider a problem in your family, indicate how it might be externalized, and speculate on the consequences.

283. Describe a "problem saturated" story or self-defeating narrative that is told in your family. How does it reflect despair, frustration, or a sense of powerlessness?

284. Is there a subjugated story hiding in the above narrative? Retell the story from this new perspective.

285. After you (as therapist) help a wife and husband to realize that her depression was related to an internalized negative narrative about woman's subordinate position in society, the woman becomes very angry, not only with her husband but with all men. For weeks she tells you that "all men are pigs." Her husband blames you and emotionally withdraws. How might narrative therapy help this couple?

286. Think of a problem you have had in your family where the attempted solutions always seemed to bring more trouble. Can you identify a "unique outcome," a time when you took some action and the problem did not get worse? What was the difference about that set of circumstances? What can you learn from the experience?

287. How would you feel if you had a problem and your therapist asked you about bringing in an "outside witness group?"

288. What would it feel like to receive a summary letter following each therapy session you attended?

289. If you had a family member reluctant to attend a family session, how would he or she respond to a "letter of invitation?"

290. Write a "redundancy letter" to a family member informing him or her that they no longer need to take the role they have been playing with you (e.g., an older sister playing mother).

291. Discuss how membership in a "league" might be useful in developing an alternative view of a problem in your family (e.g., anorexia, depression, alcoholism, chronic illness).

292. An elderly married couple along with their adult children come to you for help in coping with the elder man's provisional diagnosis of Alzheimer's disease. You are told that for his entire life, he viewed his responsibility to be to face reality directly without sugar coating anything. He says that he does not want to deny his current situation or the likelihood that soon he will longer be conscious of himself and his world, a turn of events that he understands will end with death. While you are impressed with this bravery, you also sense that the elderly man is very. How might narrative therapy help with the depression?

CHAPTER 15

Psychoeducational Models:
Teaching Skills to Specific Populations

Psychoeducation vs. Psychotherapy

293. Psychoeducational family therapy emphasizes interpersonal skills-building, a technique especially suited for dysfunctional families. Can you think of a family you know where such an approach would be the treatment of choice? Identify their problem and state your reasons for why psychoeducation might help them.

294. You visit your therapist and notice a manual on her desk from which she has been working with you and your family. What is your reaction? Explain why.

295. Following up the previous question, suppose you discover that your therapist has written the manual with a group of other professionals. Does that change your attitude?

296. One result of chronic mental illness may be seen in the streets of our cities. Where are the families of these homeless people? How would you address the problem of mentally ill homeless men and women?

297. Have you known a family where a member has been diagnosed with a chronic mental illness such as schizophrenia? What did you observe about family functioning?

298. Is your family a high EE (Expressed Emotion) family or a low EE family? If high, is the emotional expressiveness characterized by critical language? Describe and discuss the effects on you growing up.

299. Is it possible your family might seek psychoeducational help but not psychotherapy? Discuss.

300. Many family therapists affiliate themselves either with systems approaches or postmodern/narrative-oriented therapy. As a clinician, how would you feel about using psychoeducational approaches that tend to rely on empirical studies and research that systems and especially postmodernist practitioners tend to reject? Are these approaches necessarily contradictory? Explain.

301. If you embrace postmodern approaches to family therapy how would you feel if you read that ten empirically based studies show that depression can be successfully managed by applying specific research-proven techniques? Would you change your own postmodern approach? Why or why not?

Medical Family Therapy

302. Has there been a medical problem that affected the life of a member of your family? What kind of help of a psychological nature might have helped the family? The afflicted person? What kind of help did the family actually receive? Did it help? Explain.

303. Medical family therapy is an interdisciplinary team approach. From your perspective, what would be the pros and cons of this approach?

304. According to the text, "no biomedical event occurs without psychosocial consequences." Discuss this statement in reference to an experience in your family.

305. How do you imagine you would feel as a therapist working with a medical team? Explain.

Short-term Educational Programs

306. How would you feel about taking a marriage preparation course with your significant other? Why would (or wouldn't) you? What would you expect to learn?

307. Your church, mosque, or synagogue requires you to undergo one to three sessions of premarital counseling if you wish to be married there. Do you think this is a good idea or a bad one? Explain.

308. Do you know of couples in your family who could benefit from a short-term course in relationship enhancement? Would they be willing to participate? What might get in their way from attending? Explain,

309. You and your significant other arrive at a therapist's office for premarital counseling and are each handed a psychological inventory to fill out. What kind of feedback would you expect from the therapist?

310. Some ethnic groups exert considerable influence over the choice of marriage partners of its young people by matching individuals to one another or by forbidding marrying outside of the group. How does your own cultural background influence whom you might marry?

311. Would you and your significant other consider attending a marriage encounter weekend? Why or why not?

CLASS EXERCISE

Learning new patterns for resolving one's family problems may come from observing another family deal with an analogous problem. In Marriage Encounter weekends, couples have an opportunity to observe other married people attempt to solve their problems. Visit one of these programs and report back to the class on what you identify as the major change agents.

CHAPTER 16

Research on Family Assessment and Therapeutic Outcomes

312. Would you describe your role in your family of origin as more that of a therapist (actively intervening in family functioning) or a researcher (observing, classifying, and evaluating what was transpiring)? How did that earlier role influence your current interests?

313. Describe the difference between hypothesis-generating and hypothesis-testing research designs. Which would you adopt in studying family relationships?

314. Does the family therapy program your university or training institute accent research? Are you encouraged to think about your training in terms of developing research skills and incorporating them into a "research informed" clinical experience? Explain.

315. Outline a qualitative research design that makes use of multiple case studies to draw conclusions about family dysfunction.

316. How would you feel about filling out an extensive questionnaire prior to seeing a therapist with your family? Are you more or less likely to reveal privately held thoughts in writing or in front of your family?

317. Do you think that the emphasis placed by insurance companies on using empirically based research findings and how these are seen to affect clinical outcomes is a positive or negative development? Explain your position.

318. As a practicing clinician, would you agree to allow your work with a client to be examined by an outside party in the service of that party's research? Why or why not? If not, how do you think meaningful clinical research could be carried out?

Couple and Family Assessment Research

319. If your family were to come for family therapy, would you want the therapist to diagnose them? If yes, should the therapist share the diagnosis with the family? If no, why not?

320. Observe the structure of the place where you work or attend school. Would you characterize the climate as rigid or flexible, autocratic or democratic, competitive or cooperative? How does this climate affect your functioning?

321. Observe a family planning something that they will do together (go to a movie, a restaurant, or vacation destination, etc.). How much information can you gather about the power structure, communication patterns, and type of family functioning? Discuss.

322. The Circumplex model produces a family map depicting twenty-five types of couple or family relationships. Where on the map would you place your family or origin? Explain.

323. Score your family on each of the subscales of Moos' social environmental scale. What conclusions do you reach about their functioning?

324. Discuss how home-based services by a family therapist would have been received by your family of origin?

Family Therapy Process and Outcome Research

325. What do you believe are the three most important mechanisms that occur within a therapy session that stimulate change? Explain.

326. What aspect of family therapy research would you like to continue to explore? Research methodology? Theory building? Classification and assessment? Process or outcome research? Explain your position.

327. How useful is evidence-supported research in family therapy? What is its future? Defend your position.

CHAPTER 17

A Comparative View of Family Theories and Therapies

328. What have been the most important things you have learned about yourself and your family from these exercises?

329. Have you moved from an individual understanding of behavior to a systems view? If so, how have you changed your narrative about yourself? If not, what personal narrative provides the context for your individual understanding of behavior?

330. Have you attempted any new solutions as a result of your changing outlook? If so, how successful were you in bringing about a desired outcome? Be specific.

331. Discuss periods of both optimal and disruptive functioning in your family as you were growing up, and explain their occurrence in systems terms.

332. Should all therapy be short term? Why or why not?

333. Do you believe that your past experience has any bearing on your present or future? Explain.

334. Describe a time your family "got stuck" in a faulty solution to a problem. How was it explained then and how do you see it now?

335. Describe a dysfunctional marriage you have observed. Was there evidence of negativity, such as criticism, contempt, stonewalling, or defensiveness? Describe.

336. Describe an optimizing couple. How is their functioning different from the couple in the previous question?

337. Discuss from the vantage point of your personal experiences whether insight or action has been more helpful in producing desired change.

338. Identify characteristics of three different theories that strike you as being very similar to each other (for example, psychoanalytic interest in fantasy versus asking someone about future goals from different postmodern perspectives). What does this exercise tell you about the process of theory building?

339. If after having read this text you feel inclined to embrace one theory rather than the others, identify the theory and explain its appeal to you. How do you think the choice of theory influences clinical practice?

340. If you feel inclined towards a more eclectic approach that uses several theories, identify the theories and provide a rationale about how you can effectively apply them to clinical work.